YOUR KNOWLEDGE HAS VALUE

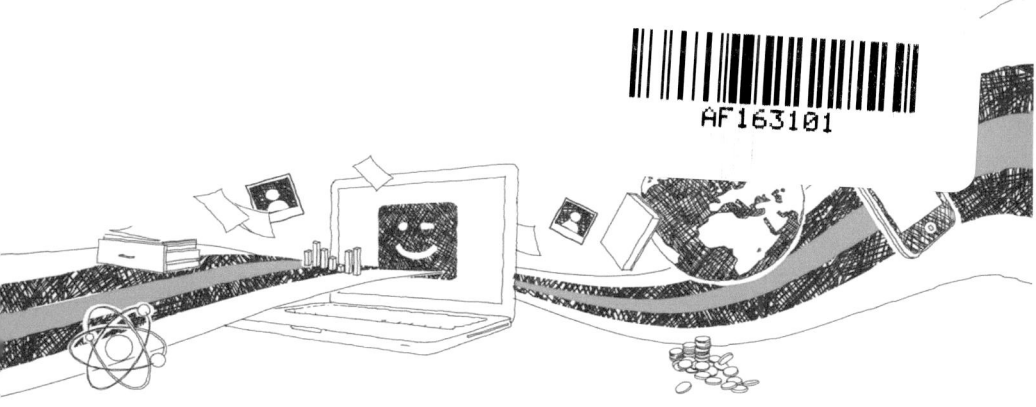

- We will publish your bachelor's and master's thesis, essays and papers

- Your own eBook and book - sold worldwide in all relevant shops

- Earn money with each sale

Upload your text at www.GRIN.com
and publish for free

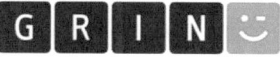

Bibliographic information published by the German National Library:

The German National Library lists this publication in the National Bibliography; detailed bibliographic data are available on the Internet at http://dnb.dnb.de .

This book is copyright material and must not be copied, reproduced, transferred, distributed, leased, licensed or publicly performed or used in any way except as specifically permitted in writing by the publishers, as allowed under the terms and conditions under which it was purchased or as strictly permitted by applicable copyright law. Any unauthorized distribution or use of this text may be a direct infringement of the author s and publisher s rights and those responsible may be liable in law accordingly.

Imprint:

Copyright © 2016 GRIN Verlag, Open Publishing GmbH
Print and binding: Books on Demand GmbH, Norderstedt Germany
ISBN: 9783668575455

This book at GRIN:

http://www.grin.com/en/e-book/381346/treating-drug-addiction-ways-to-improve-the-successful-rate-of-rehabilitation

Patrick Kimuyu

Treating drug addiction. Ways to improve the successful rate of rehabilitation

GRIN Publishing

GRIN - Your knowledge has value

Since its foundation in 1998, GRIN has specialized in publishing academic texts by students, college teachers and other academics as e-book and printed book. The website www.grin.com is an ideal platform for presenting term papers, final papers, scientific essays, dissertations and specialist books.

Visit us on the internet:

http://www.grin.com/

http://www.facebook.com/grincom

http://www.twitter.com/grin_com

Drug addiction refers to a dependence on a medication or illegal substance. Addicted people are unable to control the usage of drugs and continue using the substance despite the obvious harms associated with their behavior. Normally, drug addiction causes an intense craving for the substance making it hard for addicted people quit such behaviors. Drug addiction causes long-term consequences such physical and mental health, strained relationships, law and employments problems (Ries, Miller & Fiellin, 2009). The affected persons are encouraged to inform their doctors, support groups, friends and families in order to overcome their addiction and stay safe. Some of the commonly abused drugs include; heroin, cocaine, bhang and alcohol. The treatment option for drug addiction within medical establishments depends on various factors such the type of the drug and how its affects the user. Treatment in many medical establishments combines psychotherapy services, inpatient and outpatient programs, self-help groups and sponsors (Ries, Miller & Fiellin, 2009). The treatment options aim at reducing dependency and restore normal lives of addicts. Specifically, heroin addiction is caused by both social and psychological factors. For instance, unpleasant feelings, stress and pressure can contribute to heroin addiction. According to National Institute of Drug Abuse (2004), factors such as cultural beliefs, drug availability and lack of education deficit can also contribute to heroin addiction. In the current world, heroin addiction is treated using various drugs namely; methadone, clonidine, buprenorphine and naltrexone. This paper explores the heroin treatment methods, problems faced, the most effective method and the way to improve the successful rate of rehabilitation.

Heroin addiction can be treated by combining both the pharmacological and behavioral methods. The two procedures helps in restoring the brain normalcy resulting to reduction in criminal behaviors, increased employment rates and low spread of HIV and other diseases. When people addicted to heroin usage first quit, withdrawal symptoms such as vomiting, pain, diarrhea and nausea becomes common (Fernandez & Libby, 2013). Medication helps during the detoxification phase easing the craving and other related symptoms. This often prompts an addict to relapse. Medication targets the opioids receptors just like heroin, but they are safer and have a low likelihood of causing addiction. The mechanism of heroin pharmacological treatment can grouped into various categories namely; agonists, (which activate opioid receptors), antagonists, which blocks the receptor and partial agonists, which also activate opioid receptors but produce a smaller response (National Institute of Drug Abuse, 2004).

Methadone is an opioid agonist characterized by a slow acting action (Dean, Bilsky & Negus, 2009). Methadone is administered orally in order to reach their brain in a slow manner, reducing the "high" associated with other drug administration routes. This reduces withdrawal symptoms. Methadone has been used in treating heroin addiction since 1960 and still remains an excellent option especially to those addicts who do not responds well to other medications. Methadone is one of the most affordable drugs used in the treatment of opioid addiction (Wormer & Davis, 2012). It is vital to note the methadone is effective when carried out in special institutional and hospitals compared to clinics. Some patients are unable to travel to such clinic while other fear stigmatization. *Cochrane* reviews. The drug is only available through legalized outpatient programs which allow daily prescription to patients. Additionally, coupling methadone treatment with encouragement measures such as job skills, recreation, friendship and family lifestyles can lead to more positive results. Those patients under the methadone regime get scared of reducing their levels on fear of losing the stability effect of the drug (Marlatt & Donovan, 2007). Patients taking methadone can continue with normal life activities. Methadone has also been found to have no serious medical interaction with other regimes. This implies that patients with conditions such as cancer, diabetes, HIV/AIDS and pneumonia among other can continue with their routine medications while also using methadone treatment. However, coordination of methadone with other drugs is essential. For instance, rifampin for tuberculosis and Dilantin used for epilepsy have been found to increase the body's metabolism of methadone and thus the need raise the dosage. Methadone medications reduce the needle sharing and promiscuous behavior that can lead to HIV transmission and other diseases. This is because patients can be dosed once on a daily basis. The drug is also highly regulated (Wormer & Davis, 2012)

According to and Davis (2012), methadone causes symptoms such as fever, weight loss, diarrhea, vomiting and lacrimation among other withdrawal symptoms during the induction phase. Additionally, it is vital to titrate the initial dosage carefully since too rapid titration often produces adverse effects. In the past, respiratory depression, systemic hypotension, cardiac arrests and deaths have occurred owing to prescription of methadone. However, various studies have indicated that the majority of heroin addicts under methadone regimes successfully complete their treatment. However, this should be followed by intervention measures (Bernstein et al., 2005).

Naltrexone is another option used in treating heroin addiction. Naltrexone is an opioid antagonist, which blocks the receptor hence interfering with the rewarding effects of opioids. Researchers argue that the drug is neither sedative nor addictive hence reducing physical dependence of heroin. However, many patients find it hard in complying the treatment hence the reducing the effectiveness of the medication (Fernandez & Libby, 2013). This has forced the FDA to approve Vivitrol®, a long-acting formulation of naltrexone administered once in a month. The most common adverse effects arising from naltrexone are non-specific gastrointestinal complications such as abdominal cramping and diarrhea. FDA has also confirmed that naltrexone cause liver damage hence the need to check patients liver before prescription. Various studies have confirmed the toxicity nature of naltrexone to liver. Other studies have revealed that methadone is superior to buprenorphine (Hser et al., 2014). This indicates that the success rate is more compared to methadone on long term basis. Naltrexone treatment should be used in conjunction with counseling, family support and psychotherapy services. Researchers also argue that naltrexone activates receptors and this effect might continue even after stopping the drug usage. Additionally, increased sensitivity of receptors during medication put patients at the risk of opioid overdose. As a result, naltrexone therapy should be monitored and patient given support measures by medical practitioners. It is also vital for patient to avoid the usage of opioids during naltrexone medication. This is because can override the blockade with high dose subjecting patients to respiratory suppression and death. Other symptom of adverse effect of naltrexone includes; unusual tiredness, muscle pain, headache and trouble in sleeping (National Institute of Drug Abuse, 2004).

Buprenorphine (Subutex®) is another treatment option used in heroin treatment. Buprenorphine is partial opioid agonist capable of reducing carving without producing dangerous effects of other opioids. Evidently, Suboxone® is a formulation of buprenorphine taken sublingually or orally and is used in reducing chances of getting high by injecting the medication. The FDA approved its usage in 2002 making the drug the first medication eligible for physician prescription through Drug Addiction Treatment Act. The approval reduces the need to visit specialized clinic hence increasing access to treatment to those addicts in the dire need of the drug. It is believed that buprenorphine has a success rate of 73% to those patients who complete their treatment (Ziaaddini, Nasirian & Nakhaee, 2010). The FDA has also approved two other generics forms of Suboxone making the treatment option more affordable. Administration of Buprenorphine is manifested with adverse effects such as constipation, dizziness and headache. Patients should inform their doctors' immediately they realize such symptom in order to address them in time. Measures such as eating diet rich in fiber, exercising and drinking plenty of water should be employed to address constipation. Researchers have also found allergic reaction owing to usage of Buprenorphine (Comer, Sullivan & Walker, 2005). Patients should notify their doctors the moment they realize the presence of rashes or hives in their bodies. Additionally, few patients have reported liver problems from the medication of buprenorphine. Those patients with liver problems should notify their doctors before the commencement of medication. Bunornorphine should be contraindicated to patient with skull injury since it increases pressure in the skull worsening the condition (Fernandez & Libby, 2013).

Clonidine belongs to the class of central alpha agonists. Clonidine inhibits sympathetic outflow by decreasing the release of central catecholamine, resulting to reduced heart rate and blood pressure. More importantly, Clonidine is highly lipid soluble, readily distributes in the central nervous system and well absorbed after transdermal and oral administration. The drug is used in the treatment of withdrawal among the drug addicts. Clonidine eliminates majority of unpleasant withdrawal symptoms from patients (Ling et al par 23). The drug helps in preventing the restless leg syndrome, which is a common uncomfortable symptom associated with withdrawals. Clonidine also combats the functioning of the sympathetic nervous system making it easier for an individual to avoid withdrawal symptoms. Studies have indicated that clonidine usage among heroin addict reduces the 'pounding heart' effect common to heroin addict. Clonidine can also to treat heroin addiction since it reduces craving by a big percentage (Ling et al., 2005). Various studies have indicated that clonidine does not have long withdrawal period compared to methadone. This percentage rate is higher compared to that of naltrexone and methadone. Other studies have also found that clonidine relapses are similar to those produced by naltrexone. Based on studies from various researchers as discussed above, it can be pointed out that clonidine is the most effective drug in heroin treatment compared to the other measures. Precisely, the success rate of clonidine in detoxifying patient is estimated as 81% (Ziaaddini, Nasirian & Nakhaee, 2010).

The successful rate of rehabilitation can be improved by incorporating motivational interviewing. Motivational interviewing has been in operation since 1983, and aims at facilitating and motivating behavior change among the addicts. Normally, Motivational interviewing has a goal-client centered and goal oriented counseling services capable of eliciting behavior change. This method contradicts other approaches, which are based to health care professionals confronting addicts and imposing their point of view (Miller, 2013). This allows addict to build a rapport between the addict and the therapist hence winning trust towards the service offered. Compared non-directive counseling methods such as medication and support groups, it is more goal oriented hence capable of helping heroin addict change their behaviors for positive lives. Motivational interviewing also aims at increasing the patients' awareness by educating the addicts the potential consequences and risk of heroin usage (Henny, Miller & Rollnick, 2007). Additionally, motivational interviewing aims at envisioning a better future of addicts through encouragement. Motivational interviewing should embrace four processes namely; engaging, focusing, evoking and planning. Motivational interviewing has various advantages compared to the conventional medication since there is no risk of addiction and health complications. More importantly, it elicits critical information from the patient. The resulting information can be used to seek solutions to the addict's problems through counseling (Miller, 2013).

It is vital to note that the medical treatment discussed in this topic had certain success rate. Thus, motivational interviewing should be used along these methods so as to improve the success rate. Evidently, since addict struggle to live drug-free lives after medication and poses a high probability of going back to addiction unless given other forms of treatment, motivational interviewing should be adopted. Some people with heroin addiction might become resistant to seeking other medication on fear that the therapist might fail to understand what addictive behavior means to them (Henny, Miller & Rollnick, 2007). Addicted patients also fear being criticized while other has guiltiness on their behaviors. This might be attributed to lack of counseling and potential benefits of living a drug free life. Motivational interviewing enables therapist analyze the situation from the addicted person point of view (Bernstein et al., 2005). This method also allows the therapist to support addicts' within their capacity to ensure behavior change.

Conclusively, various studies have confirmed that clonidine is the most effective heroin treatment compared to methadone, buprenorphine and naltrexone. Heroin addiction is caused by both psychological and social factors such as stress, unpleasant feeling and pressure among other factors. Effective heroin treatment should employ the pharmacological and monitoring interviewing. Combining the two measures will aid in reducing the transmission of HIV, foster relationships and avoid unemployment. Methadone has been used in the treatment of heroin addiction since 1960. The current research indicates that patients under methadone prescription can continue with their normal life activities. Methadone is available only in legalized outpatient program. Since methadone does not cause serious drug interactions, it can be used with other regimes. Methadone causes problems such as fever, vomiting, diarrhea and respiratory depression among other effects. Naltrexone can also be used to treat heroin addiction. However, naltrexone has been found to cause gastrointestinal complications and liver damage.

FDA approved Buprenorphine for treating heroin addiction in 2002. Buprenorphine has success rate of 73% to those patients who complete their medication. Problems such as rashes, liver complication and hive can arise with the usage of Buprenorphine. Clonidine is the most effective heroin treatment drug due to its mechanism of action. It has a success rate of 81% when patient complete their medication. The success of rehabilitation can be realized by adopting motivational interviewing. This method advocates behavior change and positive living.

References

Bernstein, J., Bernstein, E., Tassiopoulos, K., Heeren, T., Levenson, S., & Hingson, R. (2005). Brief motivational intervention at a clinic visit reduces cocaine and heroin use. *Drug Alcohol Depend.* 7;77(1):49-59.

Comer, S., Sullivan, M., & Walker, E. (2005). Comparison of Intravenous Buprenorphine and Methadone Self-Administration by Recently Detoxified Heroin-Dependent Individuals. *JPET, 315*(3), 1320-1330.

Dean, R., Bilsky, E., & Negus, S. (2009). *Opiate Receptors and Antagonists: From Bench to Clinic Contemporary Neuroscience.* Berlin, Germany: Springer Science & Business Media.

Fernandez, H., & Libby, T. (2013). *Heroin: Its History, Pharmacology & Treatment.* Center City, MN: Hazelden Publishing.

Henny, H., Miller,W., & Rollnick, S. (2007). *Motivational Interviewing in the Treatment of Psychological Problems.* New York, NY: Guilford Press.

Hser, Y., Saxon, A., Huang, D., Hasson, A., Thomas, C., Hillhouse, M,…Jacobs P. (2014). Treatment retention among patients randomized to buprenorphine/naloxone compared to methadone in a multi-site trial. *Addiction, 109*(1), 79-87.

Ling W., Amass, L., Shoptaw, S., Annon, J., Hillhouse, M., Babcock, D.,…Brigham, G. (2005). A multicenter randomized trial of buprenorphine-naloxone versus clonidine for opioid detoxification: findings from the National Institute on Drug Abuse Clinical Trials Network. *Addiction, 100*(8), 1090–100.

Marlatt, G., & Donovan, D. (2007). *Relapse Prevention: Maintenance Strategies in the Treatment of Addictive Behaviors.* New York, NY: Guilford Press.

Miller, P. (2013). *Interventions for Addiction: Comprehensive Addictive Behaviors and Disorders, Volume 3.* Cambridge, MA: Academic Press.

National Institute of Drug Abuse. (2004). *Research on Heroin.* Retrieved from https://www.naabt.org/documents/HEROIN.pdf

Ries, R, Miller,S., & Fiellin, D. (2009). *Principles of Addiction Medicine.* Philadelphia, PA: Lippincott Williams & Wilkins.

Wormer, K., & Davis, D. (2012). *Addiction Treatment.* Boston, MA: Cengage Learning.

Ziaaddini, H, Nasirian, M., & Nakhaee, N. (2010). A Comparison of the Efficacy of Buprenorphine and Clonidine in Detoxification of Heroin-Dependents and the Following Maintenance Treatment. *Addict Health,* 2(1-2), 18–24. Retrieved from

http://www.ncbi.nlm.nih.gov/pmc/articles/PMC3905506/

YOUR KNOWLEDGE HAS VALUE

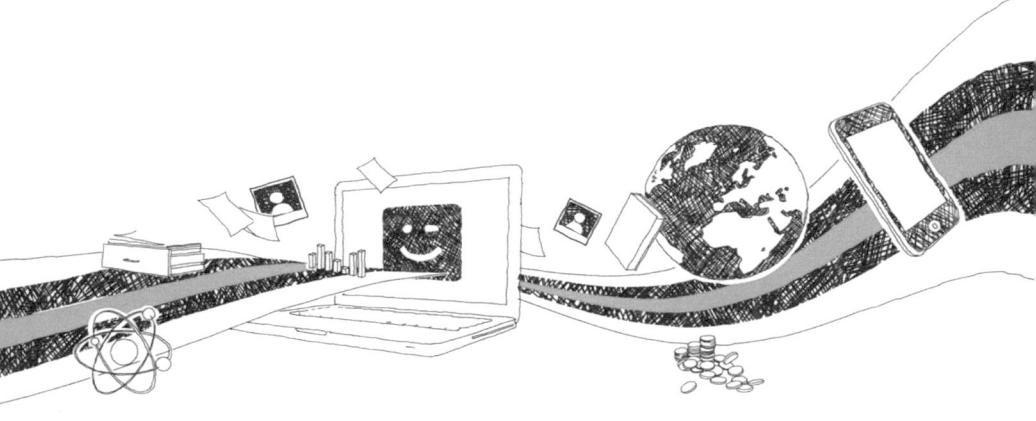

- We will publish your bachelor's and master's thesis, essays and papers

- Your own eBook and book - sold worldwide in all relevant shops

- Earn money with each sale

Upload your text at www.GRIN.com
and publish for free

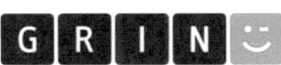